COOKBOOK FOR FIRST-TIME MOMS DURING PREGNANCY

Maria D. Johnson

TABLE OF CONTENT

INTRODUCTION

With "Cookbook for First-time Moms During Pregnancy" on a culinary voyage that honors the exquisite tapestry of pregnancy. This eBook is a thoughtfully written manual meant to accompany you on the amazing journey of becoming a mother. This compilation of recipes, thoughts, and useful advice is intended to enhance every moment of your maternity journey, whether you are enjoying the countdown to your child's arrival or navigating the postpartum phase.

Enter a world where flavor and nutrition collide, and where every meal serves as a celebration of the satisfaction that comes from feeding one's body and spirit. This book offers an abundance of culinary ideas, ranging from nutrient-rich meals to invigorating smoothies to start your day during the postpartum period.

Look past recipes to learn the tricks of sustaining

CHAPTER 1

Building a Healthy Foundation

❖ *Understanding Nutritional Needs During Pregnancy*

A woman's life transforms during pregnancy, and it is essential to provide her with a healthy diet for the growing baby as well as for her own health and growth. This chapter explores the special dietary needs that arise during pregnancy, including important nutrients, vitamins, and minerals. We examine the essential components that promote a healthy pregnancy from the first to the last trimester, arming you with the information you need to make wise food choices. Discover the value of eating a balanced diet, suggested daily intakes, and solutions for common nutritional problems. Gain the knowledge necessary to support both you and your unborn child for a smooth and healthy pregnancy experience.

❖ *Essential Nutrients for Mom and Baby*

Meeting certain dietary demands that support the growing baby's health as well as the expecting mother's is essential to ensuring a good pregnancy. The primary necessary nutrients that are vital during pregnancy are the subject of this chapter. We examine the functions of vital minerals like iron and calcium, as well as vital vitamins like D and folic acid, in promoting the fetus's growth and development and the mother's overall health. Learn about the origins of these nutrients, the suggested daily consumption, and any possible advantages. Knowing the significance of these fundamental components enables expectant moms to make educated food decisions that support a healthy pregnancy for both the expectant mother and the unborn child.

❖ *Creating a Balanced Diet Plan*

Creating a meal plan that is both nutritionally sound and well-rounded is essential to promoting a bright and healthy pregnancy. This chapter walks you through creating a nutrition plan that is balanced and catered to the unique requirements of pregnant moms. Investigate several food categories, portion management, and the importance of including a range of nutrients in your regular meals. Discover how to balance your intake of carbs, proteins, fats, vitamins, and minerals to fulfill the special needs of pregnancy. You'll find helpful hints and meal ideas to help you create a healthy, fulfilling diet that benefits your general health and the health of your infant. During this unique period of your life, embrace the road toward a health-conscious and balanced diet.

CHAPTER 2

Breakfast Delights

❖ *Energizing Smoothies and Juices*

This chapter features delicious and nourishing juices and smoothies that are meant to provide expecting mothers a quick boost of energy. Learn about a range of meals that include vital vitamins and minerals that are necessary for a healthy pregnancy in addition to tasting great. These invigorating drinks, which range from colorful fruit mixes to nutrient-rich green mixtures, are designed to promote your overall health and tackle typical pregnancy-related issues. Find out why including these cool beverages into your everyday routine is beneficial and get inspired to modify recipes to your own tastes. These revitalizing smoothies and juices provide a delicious way to feed both you and your developing baby, whether

you're searching for a quick breakfast
alternative or a refreshing pick-me-up
during the day.

❖ *Protein-Packed Breakfasts*

Choose from a variety of high-protein breakfast options designed specifically for pregnant mothers to kickstart your day. This chapter looks at tasty and filling dishes that give your body the critical protein it needs while you're pregnant. Find a variety of methods to include high-quality proteins in your morning routine, from filling breakfast bowls to revitalizing smoothies. Discover the advantages of protein for your baby's growth as well as for yourself, and try out some inventive ingredient combinations to make breakfast tasty and nourishing. These high-protein breakfast options can help you easily satisfy your increased nutritional needs throughout pregnancy by keeping you feeling satisfied, energized, and prepared to take on the day.

❖ *Healthy Grain and Fruit Options*

This chapter explicitly addresses the nutritional needs of expecting moms with regard to healthful, tasty, and nutritious breakfast options that include a range of fruits and whole grains. Discover a variety of dishes that highlight the benefits of whole grains like quinoa, whole wheat, and oats when combined with a variety of tasty fruits. These alternatives, which range from filling grain bowls to delicious parfaits, offer a good mix of important nutrients including fiber, vitamins, and antioxidants. Find out why it's so important to include these nutrients in your morning routine to promote general health while pregnant. These nutritious grain and fruit breakfast recipes, with their variety of textures and flavors, provide a lovely way to start your day while supporting your developing baby and yourself.

CHAPTER 3

Lunchtime Favorites

❖ *Nutrient-Rich Salad Bowls*

This chapter features colorful, nutrient-dense salads that are especially designed for pregnant moms. Discover a range of salad bowl dishes that will entice your palate while also offering vital vitamins and minerals that are necessary for a safe pregnancy. With their vibrant veggies, lush greens, and protein-rich additions, these salads provide a delicious blend of textures and flavors. Learn the nutritional advantages of adding a variety of items to your salads and how to make tasty, well-balanced meals that meet your heightened nutritional requirements while pregnant. These nutrient-dense salad bowls are a light and filling choice that make it simple to stick to a balanced diet while enjoying tasty and nutritious combinations.

❖ *Quick and Easy Sandwiches*

A selection of quick, nutrient-dense sandwich recipes designed to satisfy the dietary requirements of expecting moms are included in this chapter. Discover a range of quick and simple sandwich recipes that include the vital nutrients for a healthy pregnancy, from traditional combos to creative twists. For a filling and nutritious supper, look into selections with lean meats, fresh veggies, and whole-grain breads. Discover how to make sandwiches that are well-rounded by combining a variety of textures and flavors. Whether you're making a fast lunch on the run or a straightforward dinner at home, these tasty sandwich ideas provide an easy way to keep a healthy diet throughout pregnancy without sacrificing convenience or flavor.

❖ *One-Pot Pregnancy-Friendly Soups*

This chapter offers a delicious collection of filling, well-balanced one-pot soup recipes that have been carefully chosen for pregnant women. Savor satisfying bowls that offer a great balance of tastes and vital nutrients, packed with a variety of veggies, lean meats, and nutritious broths. These simple-to-make soups are ideal for pregnant women since they fulfill your increased nutritional needs without being difficult to prepare. Learn the advantages of adding a variety of ingredients to these one-pot miracles that provide a hearty and filling alternative for any dinner. These soups, which range from creative blends to comforting classics, provide a tasty and practical way to fuel you and your developing child during this unique time.

CHAPTER 4

Wholesome Dinners

❖ *Balanced Sheet Pan Meals*

This chapter examines balanced sheet pan meals that are suited to the nutritional requirements of pregnant moms, both in terms of convenience and nutrition. Learn how to prepare a range of dishes on a single sheet pan that feature a well-balanced combination of veggies, healthy grains, and meats. In addition to being simple to make, these meals provide a balanced intake of nutrients and tastes. Find out how using a variety of ingredients in sheet pan cooking may help you satisfy your increased nutritional demands while pregnant easily and with ease. From flavored fish and vivid grains to savory chicken and roasted veggies, these well-balanced sheet pan dinners provide a tasty and effective method to keep a wholesome diet while enjoying a variety of interesting and fulfilling combinations.

❖ *Nourishing One-Pot Recipes*

This chapter offers a selection of healthy one-pot dishes created to meet the unique dietary requirements of new moms. Discover an assortment of healthful and well-balanced dishes that combine easily in one pot, reducing cleaning and enhancing taste. These dishes, which range from filling casseroles and robust stews to nutrient-dense grain bowls, combine grains, veggies, and proteins to create a balanced and gratifying dinner. Experience the ease and quickness of one-pot cooking while giving vital nutrients for a healthy pregnancy first priority. Emphasizing both simplicity of preparation and nourishing content, these dishes provide a delectable choice for preoccupied expectant mothers looking for nutritious and delectable solutions for this unique occasion.

❖ *Vegetarian and Vegan Options*

This chapter is devoted to offering pregnant moms who are following a vegetarian or vegan diet a variety of nutritious balanced alternatives. Discover a variety of mouthwatering dishes that highlight the wealth of plant-based foods and provide vital nutrients for a healthy pregnancy. These dishes provide a range of tasty and filling alternatives, from nutrient-dense veggies to plant sources high in protein. Find out which nutrients are most important for vegetarian and vegan diets during pregnancy, and receive ideas for preparing meals that have a variety of tastes and textures. These recipes are great for vegetarians and vegans who wish to experiment more with plant-based diets or who just want to eat a healthier diet for themselves and their developing child.

CHAPTER 5

Snack Smart

❖ *Power-Packed Pregnancy Snacks*

In this chapter, explore a selection of energizing and nutrient-dense snacks specifically tailored for expectant mothers. Discover a variety of delicious options that provide quick bursts of energy while addressing the unique nutritional needs of pregnancy. From protein-packed bites to wholesome trail mixes and flavorful fruit combinations, these snacks are designed to keep you fueled and satisfied between meals. Learn about the importance of incorporating a mix of nutrients into your snacks to support both your well-being and the growth of your baby. Whether you're combating cravings or simply looking for convenient and nourishing snacks, these power-packed options offer a tasty and health-conscious solution for the snacking preferences of expectant moms.

❖ *DIY Trail Mix and Energy Bites*

Explore the world of homemade snacks in this chapter, where you will learn how to make your own trail mix and energy bites that are perfect for expecting women. Discover how to put together a customized trail mix that offers a pleasing combination of flavors and textures and fits your taste preferences by combining a variety of nuts, seeds, dried fruits, and other wholesome components. Explore recipes for energy bites as well. These are little, potent snacks that provide a rapid energy boost and vital minerals. Learn about the advantages of these individualized snacks, which can help with energy levels and certain nutritional requirements connected to pregnancy. These homemade trail mix and energy bite recipes provide a tasty and nutritious option for when you're on the road or in need of a quick and filling pick-me-up.

❖ *Healthy Sweet Treats*

Savor guilt-free pleasures with this chapter's assortment of nutritious sweets that are ideal for nursing moms. Discover how to satiate your sweet needs while getting the vital elements you need for a healthy, balanced diet during pregnancy. These sweets, which range from fruit-infused pleasures to naturally sweetened desserts, provide a healthy substitute for typical sugary munchies. Find inventive methods to include nutrient-dense components to your baked goods, such as fruits, nuts, and whole grains. Discover the advantages of selecting healthier sweet alternatives when pregnant and get ideas for scrumptious and nutritious sweets. These nutritious sweet snacks are a pleasant complement to your pregnant journey, whether you're pampering yourself or commemorating a special event.

CHAPTER 6

Hydration and Mocktails

❖ *Staying Hydrated During Pregnancy*

Staying hydrated is essential to keeping a pregnancy healthy. This chapter discusses the significance of maintaining proper hydration and provides advice on how to satisfy your increased fluid requirements during this unique period. Discover the health advantages of water and fun ways to flavor it with fruits and herbs. Learn the value of additional hydrating drinks and how to make wise decisions to promote both your developing baby's and your own well-being. Discover entertaining methods to stay as hydrated as possible throughout your pregnancy, from herbal teas to cool infused water dishes. During this significant and transformational time, embrace the benefits of enough hydration for your energy, digestion, and general health.

❖ *Refreshing Non-Alcoholic Beverage Recipes*

This chapter offers a selection of delicious, non-alcoholic drink recipes that will help you stay hydrated and rejuvenated during your pregnancy. Find tasty substitutes for typical alcoholic beverages, such as fruity mocktails and herbal infusions. Try these dishes that will not only make you feel better, but will also provide you and your unborn child a healthy dose of vitamins and minerals. Discover how to blend fresh fruits, herbs, and other healthful ingredients to create cool beverages. These recipes for non-alcoholic beverages offer a delicious and health-conscious way to enjoy a broad variety of refreshing drinks during your pregnancy journey, whether you're searching for a mocktail to celebrate memorable occasions or a calming herbal infusion to relax.

CHAPTER 7
Managing Cravings

❖ Understanding Pregnancy Cravings

This chapter explores the diverse reasons that lead to these distinct and frequently strong cravings for certain meals, delving into the fascinating realm of pregnant cravings. Find more about the hormonal and physiological changes that occur during pregnancy and how they may affect desires. You may also want to consider the possible emotional and psychological effects. Learn about common cravings—from savory and salty to sweet and unexpected combinations—and their potential causes. Learn how to effectively control and satiate your desires so that you may maintain your nutritional requirements while occasionally indulging in a pleasure. Gaining knowledge about the intricacies of pregnancy cravings will enable you to make wise decisions and manage this part of your journey with mindfulness, resulting in a balanced and joyful pregnant experience.

❖ Healthy Alternatives to Satisfy Cravings

Discover wholesome and fulfilling ways to enjoy and deal with pregnant cravings in a way that is health-conscious in this chapter. Find a range of healthful choices that will satisfy your desires while also providing vital nutrients for a well-balanced pregnancy diet. Learn how to create conscious food choices that satisfy your cravings for certain flavors without sacrificing your nutritional needs, whether they be crunchy snacks or sweet delights. Look for inventive ways to replace conventional meals that cause cravings, as well as dishes that provide healthier options. Gain the ability to control your urges in a way that promotes both your health and your child's best possible growth. You may balance satiating your cravings and keeping a balanced diet throughout this transforming moment by adopting these healthy options.

CHAPTER 8

Special Occasions

❖ *Celebrating Milestones with Pregnancy-Friendly Recipes*

This chapter includes a variety of delicious and well-balanced meals to help you celebrate significant occasions throughout your pregnancy journey. These recipes are intended to bring a festive touch to these happy occasions, such as pregnancy announcements, gender reveal parties, or other noteworthy occasions. Discover inventive pregnancy-friendly recipes that suit a range of dietary needs and palates. These dishes, which range from appetizers and main meals to mouthwatering desserts, are created with taste and nutrition in mind. Discover how to prepare a delicious and health-conscious meal for your developing child, your loved ones, and yourself. Savor delectable cuisine to commemorate each milestone, which not only signifies the celebration but also adds to a fulfilling and pleasurable pregnant experience.

❖ *Baby Shower Treats and Menus*

This chapter offers a variety of delicacies and cuisines that are appropriate for pregnant women in an effort to make the baby shower experience enjoyable and unforgettable. Discover a range of savory and sweet alternatives to suit a variety of dietary requirements and tastes. These dishes, which range from lovely sweets to appealing appetizers, are designed to commemorate the impending baby's arrival in style. Find inventive ideas for themed baby shower dinners that will enhance the festive and cheerful ambiance while also pleasing the palate. Discover how to organize and carry out a baby shower that ensures a fun and health-conscious celebration while giving careful concern to the dietary requirements of the expecting mother. Make the baby shower a memorable event by arranging these mouthwatering and eye-catching dishes and snacks.

CHAPTER 9

Postpartum Nutrition

❖ *Nutrient-Rich Meals for the Postpartum Period*

Making healthy, nourishing meals that are especially suited to the postpartum stage is the main topic of this chapter. Learn how to restore vital vitamins and minerals that may have been lost after delivery with these nutrient-dense meal options. These meals, which range from hearty soups and stews to protein-rich foods, are carefully chosen to promote healing and supply the energy required during this period of transition. Find out what foods to eat after giving birth, especially those that help women recuperate and nurse. Examine doable strategies for food preparation and planning to help make the postpartum phase more nutrient-sound and manageable. You may improve your general health and guarantee a good start to the postpartum journey by making nutrient-rich meals a priority.

❖ *Supporting Breastfeeding with the Right Foods*

This chapter explores the vital role that diet plays in assisting nursing moms. Investigate a range of foods that can enhance breastfeeding and supply the vital nutrients required by the infant and mother. Find out about the special meals that should be consumed throughout the breastfeeding phase in order to improve the quantity and quality of your milk. Find a variety of mouthwatering, lactation-friendly dishes that will make mealtimes fun while providing the nursing mother with the best possible nourishment. Learn the value of eating well-balanced meals, staying hydrated, and consuming essential nutrients like omega-3 fatty acids. You can fuel yourself and provide your baby the finest nutrition possible during the nursing journey by including the correct items in your diet.

CHAPTER 10

Quick Tips and Tricks

❖ *Time-Saving Kitchen Hacks*

In order to make cooking and food preparation easier during the hectic time of motherhood, this chapter is devoted to useful and effective kitchen hacks. Learn clever tricks and methods to streamline the cooking process, increase productivity, and save time. Make your time in the kitchen more manageable with these tips, which range from smart ingredient prep to batch cooking techniques. Find out how to streamline processes, keep your kitchen neat, and need less cleanup. These practical tips for the kitchen will help you manage the demands of parenthood while still enjoying tasty and nutritious meals, regardless of whether you're a new mother or just searching for methods to cook more efficiently.

❖ *Preparing Meals in Advance*

The advantages of meal planning to save time and expedite the cooking process—particularly during hectic times like motherhood—are the main topic of this chapter. Examine efficient methods for organizing and cooking meals ahead of time to make sure you always have wholesome, delectable selections on hand. Learn how to make a range of meals in a single cooking session, from freezer-friendly recipes to bulk cooking. Discover how to plan your meals for the coming week or month, select recipes that are easy to prepare, and properly store food. You can make cooking easier on a daily basis, lessen stress, and guarantee that your family has access to healthy and easy food alternatives by making meal preparation in advance a habit.

❖ *Budget-Friendly Options*

The purpose of this chapter is to examine affordable methods and recipes that will enable you to keep a balanced, healthful diet without going over budget. Make the most of your grocery budget by learning how to choose inexpensive items, use wise shopping strategies, and create cost-effective meal plans. This chapter offers helpful advice on making cost-effective meals that are both tasty and healthful, from inexpensive cupboard staples to adaptable foods that can be used for several meals. Discover how to use cost-effective substitutes without sacrificing flavor or nutrition, shop wisely, and reduce food waste. You may attain a well-balanced and economical approach to feeding your family and yourself by implementing these money-saving strategies into your meal planning.

CONCLUSION

We would like to take this opportunity to offer our sincere congratulations on your pregnancy as you get to the end of this cookbook. It's an amazing accomplishment to embrace the life-changing experience of motherhood, and we applaud your commitment to nurturing your developing child as well as yourself.

I hope the recipes, advice, and insights included within these pages help make your pregnancy a tasty, healthy, and happy experience. Keep in mind that every meal is an opportunity to nurture both you and your child, fostering happy and meaningful moments.

I hope your journey into parenting is easy and lovely. I hope you have a lot of love, health, and the simple joys of cooking and eating wholesome meals with your expanding family. Once more, congratulations and best wishes for the fascinating voyage that lies ahead!